Yoga:

2021 Guide For Healing Strengthening and Stress Relief.

Yoga

ISBN: 9798709790292

CONTENTS

Introduction 4

What is Yoga? What does it mean? 9

What is Mudra? 21

How to practice and progress 24

Develop the meditation practice of your child 63

Don't wait for immediate results 65

Seek professional assistance 68

Help on the Road 72

Yoga is about mental and physical health 82

Conclusion 87

Introduction

Have you ever wondered what is yoga? What is the source of yoga? Where did yoga begin? What is the "ultimate truth?" What is yoga "stotra?" And when, where and how did yoga start?

What is yoga? What is yoga?

The early epic Sanskrit poem, the Arthashastra 250 BCE, discusses the factors that contribute to the production of spiritual life, the management of mind and emotions. It was from this text that the word "yuga" originated and which means the union or completion of form, matter and energy, which can be traced to very old Indian scriptures.

And who is yogi? And who the yogi?

The Yogi is an ego-freed soul, based on clear, harmonious thinking and direct experience of the essence of the Self, the divine spark which animates the universe.

And what's the "last truth?"

Yoga means union and completion of form, matter and energy. The idea of "Yoga" can be directly translated into the state of being which is characterized by a state of mental tranquility, meditative stillness and direct experience of the divine.

When did you start yoga?

Yoga has been practiced by humans since the Vedic era (2500 BCE) and by our human ancestors since time immemorial. It is said that the wise Agastya discovered yoga in India around 3000 BCE.

How did yoga become?

A very simple account of the beginning of yoga is as follows:

This Yogi had realized the purpose of all the devas, gods, planets and all the ancient Gods. He realized that the Deity, (Shakti) can only come into manifestness through the preparation of his body and mind. The human body and mind, a formless energy, is the reserve of all the energies of creation. The body is the temple of this energy manifested.. But if these activities are not controlled or directed, the accumulated energy is released into the physical body that is wastes, loses or transfers to the mind, which can be mistaken, intense or disruptive.

The yogi realized that the mind should be put in its proper place to control the body. If the mind is not organized, the consciousness of the body cannot be regulated. The body and mind are closely connected and the effects of the body will also affect the mind. So, it is important to be in a state of mental tranquility.

It is very important for us to understand the concept of yoga in the context of science, because modern science has concluded that many kinds of consciousness exist, we refer to them as 'fields of consciousness' and we can have some sort of experience similar to 'Spiritual perception' in this field of consciousness because consciousness is projected from a space of science..

It's not to say that the body is not part of our collective consciousness. Rather it is important to know that there are many ways to experience our consciousness and that the field of consciousness is not the same as our own body.

What is Yoga? What does it mean?

Let us look at the word 'yoga' and how the practice was described.

Yoga is a system of practice and meditation.

Yoga means a union; that is, a union between mind, body and spirit. It means the harmony in the form of man.

Yoga is to be practiced to reach the "kingdom of God."

Yoga, including Indian Himalayas, can be practiced everywhere.

Yoga can create a physical and mental relaxation equivalent to a mountain holiday.

Yoga is a spiritual practice that helps to connect the mind with the body and the body with the spirit.

It must be practiced by all to achieve a better quality of life.

Yoga is considered to be a good human being's five essential practices.

Yoga is the union of the principles of men and women in a consciousness system.

Yoga can be practiced in all levels of the human body consciousness.

Yoga has unlimited benefits: better sleep, lower blood pressure, better digestion, better concentration, better immune system, better physical health, less stress, better health, deeper meditation, increased concentration, control over oneself, increased creativity, and inspiration.

In order to learn this old practice you have to develop discipline and patience. In order for results to be achieved, you will need the power to stay the course, and the ability to fully commit yourself to the practice. If you are not willing to fully engage, do not follow Yoga.

You'll need to find a teacher that you can trust and guide you on your journey. You will also need to dedicate time to meditation and learn how to get your mind to be at ease. The most important thing is to believe in the power of practice and repetition and not give up on the journey of self-realization.

I think it's a great time to teach you and your pupils a yoga course. I know from my education that quality and compassionate training in this field are necessary.

The many advantages of yoga

The many advantages of yoga

Columbia, SC (WOLO) — The trend towards hot yoga has an important effect on the gym.

Yoga-studio owner Tricia Peters says that because of all the health benefits the main reason that yoga was so popular is.

The hot yoga trend is the result of the 90-minute hot yoga session Bikram.

They are held in a room heated to about 120 degrees.

There are many benefits to yoga – improve flexibility, increase energy and regulate emotions. But it can be difficult to achieve health benefits – there is more than one way to bring your body together in the correct way.

When the weather is cool and you want to be active or warm from within, yoga is a great way to take your mind and body to new places.

Heidi Davis, owner of the Scottsdale Yoga Center and the Run or Dye, said lifelong practice is to align your mind and mind with your spirit.

"It's all about building on what you know and building on what you want to feel," Davis said. "It's the use of what we know and what we work with."

Davis regularly teaches yoga in the valley. She said you'll work with the energy of the universe when you do yoga. This is how you connect with your inner being and make things you want to do in your life.

"This is a way to improve your healthy lifestyle," said Davis.

Davis said it can be easy to get results once you know how to do Yoga. You need to stay consistent with the practice and learn from your experience, she said.

"I think it comes back to being attentive," Davis said. "If you listen to yourself and your body and pay attention, I think you'll make a great deal of progress.

Davis has added that it is important to find the right teacher and be careful about what they teach you.

The way the body moves can be soothing and curing. When you're in a different line-up, a deeper sense of healing is possible, Davis said.

"I think it helps free everything that you hold within, and in every way it is helpful," Davis said. "It benefits the body and the mind and the spirit."

To download the free azfamily mobile app, click/tap here.

As a culture, we must begin with addressing cultural appropriation if we look today at the causes of separation in yoga.

Current yoga cultures are a treasure trove for all from secret language, healing, spiritual goals, and spiritual history. we are fortunate to be able to immerse ourselves deeply in the roots of who we are and how, over time, our own perspectives, beliefs, experiences and issues have shaped us.

However, since these profoundly rich traditions have been there for so long, there is a tendency to take everything for granted.

Modern yoga cultures are a treasure trove of secret languages, healing practices, spiritual purposes and spiritual history.

One instance I have found is a class I taught last summer that focuses on neuro-linguistic programming, which has now been translated into several languages and which have influenced thousands of people worldwide.

As CD-designer who was with me, I had the opportunity to share everything I had learnt on my journey to develop a CD. However, I also had an extensive experience, study and experience. So the process of designing this DVD was not just an exciting challenge, but also an opportunity to share what I learned during my course development.

As a culture, when we look today at the causes of yoga division, we must start by addressing cultural appropriation.

I do not advise to hold on to old knowledge, to pretend that all that is sacred is not appropriate, or that only the official, published yoga texts are true.

I support everyone's right to ask questions and to seek answers in accordance with the instructions for teachers. We continually redefine our understanding of yoga and spiritual practice.

It is more than acceptable and ethical to respect the histories and traditions of those who have been practicing yoga and teaching mercy and tolerance for centenaries. We must start by recognizing that ascertaining our sources of information, adapting them to our circumstances and sharing our findations in a manner appropriate, useful and meaningful for our communities is the aim of

We are responsible for raising conscience and advancing what we are most enthusiastic about, for those who have chosen to teach and to share our understanding of the wisdom we have learned and help to move modern yoga into the modern world. And regardless of our affiliations, we must try to act on the highest moral and ethical standards.

Treating old versus new culture is an uncomfortable environment, and those of us who are privileged to get there need to become more aware of the differences, intentions, motivations and contributions.

So I hope that when we speak about the kind of cultural appropriation in yoga we become aware of the deeply linked and deeply vulnerable systems created in the name of yoga, and that we can begin to build the space for confidence, that leads us to explore, expand and develop towards greater freedom and health.

Whats mudra and how to practice it. Here are some best breathing techniques.

What is Mudra?

Mudra is a Sanskrit word for a dot placed on the forehead, a circular hand gesture, etc. The meaning of Mudra is expression or sign or movement.

Mudra is a way to improve concentration and meditation by focusing on an object. It will help you focus and bring more awareness in your body and mind.

Mudra is supposed to be done while meditating, some believe Mudra could also be done while praying or during meditation. You need to be strong to do it effectively.

If you want to learn Mudra, here are some easy steps to follow.

Steps to learn Mudra:

Identify what Mudra you need to learn.

Find an object or material that could be in your meditation space.

Use some kana (scroll) paper and a pen to draw out the desired Mudra.

Begin to observe, while you do the Mudra, your breath. What happens to your breath as you do the Mudra?

Do a short meditation session. (You dont need to do it long.)

Using visualisation technique, if you wish, you can visualize that the Mudra you are drawing is like your palm. Let it hang at the bottom of your palm. It is like a long finger or thumb. With the inner part of your palm, keep your thumb at the center and rest your pointer finger on your inner third (just below the knuckle). Keep your ring finger and pinky at the outer part of the thumb. In other words, keep your Mudras long arm hang in the center, just below your palm. Try to put the Mudra away after doing a few of them. You can do this when you have some free time or if you practice it for more than 5 minutes a day, it will be more likely to work.

How to practice and progress

In my experience, a little bit of meditation and visualization is enough for a good meditation. At first you may not notice much change, but gradually you will notice the difference. You can see the results after doing some Mudra for more than a few minutes.

Before I practice meditation, I try to visualize some living organisms. Once you find some animals or plants or insects, you can choose one and focus on it. Try to remember that your focus on the Mudra is like a small appendage, your thumb can be like the eye or the penis, the middle finger is like the eyelid. Try to concentrate on the way it moves.

So dont worry too much about where to draw your Mudra. Instead try to use visualization and some simple meditation to master it.

Enjoy your meditation with some of the best breathing techniques.

How to start learning yoga ? I want to find a good yoga teachers. Criterias to find a good teacher are: Is the teacher specialized in your style of yoga ?

Is the teacher passionate about this type of yoga ?

Is the teacher very efficient and always on time.

Is the teacher humble and never looks down on his/her students.

Is the teacher willing to talk to you when you are having doubts and problems.

Is the teacher accepting of new people to his/her yoga ?

Is the teacher is not very talkative to his/her students

What do you consider the attributes of a good teacher ? Be attentive, compassionate, humble, timely, good communicator and flexible. Also you must have a good yoga body. Thats why it is a perfect combination. But on the next to last point I want to let you to ask yourself what you think is the character of a good teacher. Because the worst characteristic is the bad attitude. If he is talking to you like a spoiled child or he is thinking that he knows more than you. That's why to work with the right teacher you have to find one with a good balance.

I want to know the best way how to start learning Yoga ? I want to find a good teacher. How can I start? Is there a way ?

First of all if you are living in a big city you have the possibility to see a good yoga school in a form of speciality or branch. But if you are living in a small town the very best option for you is to meet your yoga teacher. And you must not hesitate to pay for a monthly or a yearly subscription. The cost of one class is 500 dollars. And it's 100 dollars per month for you to visit him. The last but not least thing to know is that in the yoga world there is no "perfect" teacher. There is no perfect person. What's important is to find someone that works for you. You can practice a lot with one person, but you can't do it with many.

Have you ever been the teacher of the first time? Can you recall your first day in front of a classroom with students? What was the first thing you did ?

The first day in front of a classroom is very difficult for a teacher. They don't know what will happen during the day. The students will be the main topic of your attention all day long. It's not easy to control the nervous energy in the classroom. During my first day in front of a classroom I started my yoga teaching by standing in front of the blackboard and I started to speak about the structure of the asanas. I would like to give you the structure that I use to explain the asanas to my students during a yoga class :

The first things you should remember is to visualize yourself balancing in yogic poses. Then you need to focus on these balancing asanas. The core of your Ashtanga yoga practice. The daily practices of asanas and pranayama. The correct mind, the techniques for finding the breath. It's good to practice the four yogic asanas each day. If you don't find the motivation to do this then I recommend to mix these four asanas in a yoga practice. It gives you the energy and motivation to do daily practices. And the main thing is the complete concentration of the mind. Focus on the breath. On your awareness. This is what can help you to perform a beautiful and unique yoga practice every day. If you have the feeling that you don't have the power to concentrate, but in one part of your mind you can see that your body is changing and that you are balancing you have problems. When the breathing is taking place in your throat or you can only concentrate on the breathing. Focus your mind on the breath.

Now I am leaving you with the last question. Please let me know what your expectations are for the future and what are your plans for this year ?

I am very happy because my plans are in place. I am preparing a project for this year to write a book and a blog. In spring I plan to have a trip to India and England to stay in my Ashtanga teachers house. I already spoke with him and he is going to help me to have a website with his experience and knowledge. We are going to write a lot about Ashtanga yoga, it's nice to share with you all the secrets of the Ashtanga yoga. This is very useful for everyone.

So, this is the end of my last interview of the year !

I want to wish everyone a happy and safe new year, a year full of Ashtanga yoga, meditation, love, money and health !

I hope you will follow my blog and will like my updates in the future! Thank you for having supported me throughout this year. A big big hug and a kiss for all of you and I hope to see you next year !
Poses we should all be practicing on the regularregardless of level and whichever

shiny, new goal pose weve had tunnel vision on.

Focusing on connecting your breathing and moving your body in slow and steady movements has shown to not only produce a deeper and more relaxed state of mind, but has also helped increase blood circulation in the body, relax the mind, and have an overall positive effect on physical strength and functionality.

Being a student of yoga, I often find myself practicing different postures when I dont have time to attend a class. Yoga involves learning how to maintain your breath, follow your body through complex movements, and having each and every part of your body is activated.

This weekly series aims to document the poses that we love to perform, whether in a studio or in our living rooms. Today well start with the set of 10 serenity poses, which are both physically and mentally relaxing for anyone to practice.

Serenity Pose #1 – Half Pigeon Pose

This pose is relaxing and gentle for anyone to practice, and a huge component to any number of meditation or self-care rituals. Make sure to keep the head in line with the spine throughout the entire pose, and dont forget to breathe throughout the process.

Serenity Pose #2 – Shavasana

Another incredibly restorative pose, I love this position to help me relax before bed, anytime of the day. Asana practice, or yoga, has been found to reduce anxiety and relieve pain in many cases.

If your mind feels like a whirlwind or your body is aching, this is a great serene position to take a breather.

Serenity Pose #3 – Iyengar Dandasana

This pose is very beneficial for anyone to practice when balancing, which is common in yoga. As you balance yourself, inhale and exhale slowly, making sure to exhale as you push back up.

Try to make sure that your hands and arms are behind your body as you engage your back. The more you breathe and relax during the transition, the less likely youll have any concerns about falling.

Serenity Pose #4 – Locust Pose

This calming pose is something you can do anywhere in the world. Locust is done slowly with the arms folded, feeling weightless. The exhale out of your mouth should feel smooth, while inhaling should come from your belly.

For those of you with an affinity for movement, try to start to roll your shoulders down toward your chest as you reach your arms down, pressing your palms against the mat.

Serenity Pose #5 – Downward Facing Dog Pose

This very intimate, restorative pose is one of the most popular asanas in all of yoga. It is very inspiring and relaxing for many people, and is just as beautiful in its different variations. It is a wonderful prop for many women and men to practice with as well, as it can be difficult for people with joint pains to contort their bodies into a pose such as Savasana.

Begin by sitting up tall, leaning against your feet, hips, and knees. Reach your arms down, placing your palms flat on the floor and fingers to reach the floor. Rotate your shoulders to bring the elbows out as close to your feet as you can. This will help you get a deeper stretch in your spine and shoulders.

Reach your hands up to the sky, and slowly lower yourself to the floor, with your body as straight as possible.

Serenity Pose #6 – Childs Pose

This pose is a wonderful option for anyone who finds sitting in a lot of yoga studios to be tiring and uncomfortable. In this asana, youll feel as though youre almost falling asleep. This position is meant to be relaxing, for sure, but its also intended to get your heart rate and breathing regulated.

Try to keep your hips hip-width apart and you will be able to lie comfortably on your back. Begin by slowly moving your arms in circles as you exhale and inhale, to make sure to get the feeling of this pose correctly. This is a very comfortable position that can often feel like youre falling asleep, but that is entirely normal.

Serenity Pose #7 – Utthita Parsvakonasana

This is one of my favorite, most restorative poses, as it is wonderful to improve flexibility, relieve stress, and get all of your muscles moving and working together. Utthita parsvakonasana is the final pose of your sun salutations sequence, and it is a very powerful one for your inner-muscles. It feels great to let your muscles fall into each other, and we always want our bodies to feel good. Try to bring your feet and knees to your hands, fingers facing forward and pointing upward.

Youll want to start out in the Viparita Karani or bow pose, or two people could alternate, but you dont have to do either one for this pose. Slowly rotate your body back to full extension, and gently bring your head down and straight to the ground. Dont forget to inhale and exhale, and you will be amazed by how nice it feels!

Serenity Pose #8 – Ardha Matsyendrasana

If you are prone to back pain or cannot lay on your back comfortably, this is a lovely stretch. This asana is excellent for general back flexibility, and many students find it helps with reducing tension in their lower back.

Begin by rolling to your left, away from your body. Your body should form a straight line, with your elbows at the sides of your body, hands flat on the mat, and feet together, in line with the feet. Place the palms of your hands on the floor.

Keep your lower back high and chest open. This will feel like you are on a roller coaster, and you may feel slightly nauseous as your body works to raise you up in the air. Your hands will begin to lift higher and higher, and then your body will fall back down to the floor, sliding your feet together behind you.

Notice the different sensations you will feel, and feel how it opens up your body. A nice breath after each movement will help you relax your body and let your muscles do their work.

Serenity Pose #9 – Ustrasana

Many yogis find that the last two poses in the sun salutation are helpful in decreasing tension and improving flexibility in their shoulders, back, and chest.

As Ustrasana, you will feel a stretch in the front of your shoulders, as well as a stretch in your back. Try to stay in your hips, and raise your arms up to touch your elbows to the sky. A deep inhale and exhale are great for this asana, as they help release tension and allow the body to move in the right way.

Serenity Pose #10 – Uttanasana

Try to stay in this asana for as long as you can, and bring your hips forward as you move your body up to your hands. This is a good stretching pose for many of our students, and will help loosen up any tight muscles in your back.

Serenity Pose #11 – Vrksasana

You will now be lying with your legs outstretched to the side, and this pose is good for relieving back tension, working on stability, and getting the muscles moving and working together.

Begin by folding your legs into cross-legged position, and then slowly bring your feet back to the floor. Remember to breathe here, and notice how your breathing changes as your body is manipulated into this position. Breathe in through your nose, and as you exhale, move your hips from side to side, getting those muscles moving and working together.

Do not over-think this pose, as this can be a very relaxing and restful pose, especially for those with shoulder or back pain.

Serenity Pose #12 – Jayavakasana

In this beautiful yogic pose, you will be lying on your back, legs spread out to the side, hands on the floor, feet pointed forward. Try to bring your head down to the floor, and follow these steps:

Take a deep breath as you breathe out of your nose.

Stomach in, find the angle and alignment that feels most comfortable, and then slowly lift your body up.

Stay steady in the pose, and stay relaxed.

Serenity Pose #13 – Anjaneyasana

Close your eyes, inhale deeply, and gently move your hips back to the center. As you exhale, bring your hands back to the floor, and stay still. The more you stay still, the easier this pose will feel. Try to breath deeply in through your nose, and then exhale through your mouth.

Serenity Pose #14 – Supta Baddha Konasana

Begin in the same way as you did before, but this time, use your feet to lift your hips off the ground a bit. Raise your hands to meet your hips, and slowly take your hips forward into Supta Baddha Konasana.

To keep your hands on the floor, start to lift them slightly up and to the sides of your head as you lift your hips. Bring your palms down to the mat, and relax.

Serenity Pose #15 – Paschimottanasana

In this very easy pose, you will move from standing on one foot to the other, with your arms stretched out to the side.

Wiggle your feet a bit, and then bend your knees to lower your body onto the floor. Use your hands to help pull your legs up into this pose, and then bring them back down.

Serenity Pose #16 – Urdhva Mukkha Svanasana

Raise your hands above your head, and your knees back to your chest.

As you lift your hips, bring your knees back, and lift your hips, too.

Continue to lift your hips and bring them back down, lifting your knees to the opposite side.

Serenity Pose #17 – Sarvangasana

Close your eyes, take deep breaths, and move your hands to the sides of your head. You will now be lying with your arms stretched above your head, with your hands reaching as far as they can toward the ceiling.

Slowly lower your torso onto the floor, extending your arms toward the floor in front of you, and then straighten your legs.

Serenity Pose #18 – Vrksasana

From this position, move your arms behind your head, and then stretch out your arms to the sides of your head.

As you do this, move your arms and arms back, and then lift your torso up, coming down slowly to rest on your hands and knees.

Relax into this pose, and breathe.

Serenity Pose #19 – Vrksasana (Downward Dog)

Reach your hands to the side of your head, fingers pointing down, and then bring your palms to the floor.

Bring your feet back into Urdhva Mukkha Svanasana, keeping your hands in a 90-degree angle on the floor.

Now, come down, come down, and bring your arms back into Urdhva Mukkha Svanasana.

Rest in Vrksasana for 10 breaths.

Then, come back up to Sarvangasana. Repeat.

Try again, and keep experimenting with poses as you become more comfortable with them.

If at first you don't succeed, try again.

#2: Get Physical

Regular physical activity is an important aspect of achieving tranquility.

It can also help to strengthen your body so you can better cope with the stresses and strains of everyday life.

Activity can help you achieve mental balance.

When you're feeling a bit stressed, a small walk outside can help.

#3: Look at a View

Connecting to nature is an easy way to find inner peace.

There's plenty of sights and sounds to look at outside that can make you happy, which is a big reason why you should do it!

Whether it's the blue sky, the bright flowers, or even a playground, connecting with nature can bring you some peace of mind.

#4: Paint or Draw

Forget thinking about the meaningless things in life and just go somewhere quiet and do something creative!

Pick a canvas or pencil and paper, or even a tablet, and take a walk or head to the park.

A regular practice of drawing, painting, or writing is a good way to channel your creativity, and it's a great way to relieve stress, too.

#5: Meditate

You can meditate in so many different ways.

Some people use guided meditations, but the following 5 tips can help anyone calm down and feel the effects of calm:

Check out a guided meditation app. They are free and easy to download and use. Make sure you take regular breaks during your meditation to re-group and recharge. Don't let your mind stray. Try to stay in the present moment at all times. Stop thinking about something trivial like whether you should get a new laptop or watch a movie instead.

#6: Take Time for Yourself

Sometimes it can be helpful to step away from your busy schedule and take some time to relax and enjoy some downtime.

Head to the bathroom and have a good cry.

Talk to your significant other or best friend about the stress that you're feeling.

Eat a full meal, perhaps with a glass of wine.

Stress can lead to overeating, but at least this way, you'll feel satisfied without eating too much.

#7: Exercise

Exercise is one of the best ways to get out some of that stress.

And for anyone who's just starting out on a fitness journey, this is another key step in becoming calmer.

I find exercise also brings with it a sense of community, and you'll often find a few of my fellow yogis getting in a sweat in the mornings.

#8: Buy a Book

Sometimes you need to make time to escape reality and read a good book.

The books that I find the most relaxing and enjoyable are ones that are insightful and can inspire and motivate me to be better.

So whatever type of book you're into, pick it up and read a few pages to start improving your mental health.

#9: Read the Sivananda Meditation Book

Sivananda is one of the greatest yogis of our time.

His book, Guide to Modern Meditation is a great way to learn some great meditation techniques.

Read the book and see if it can help you relieve some of that stress.

#10: Keep a Journal

Journaling is a great way to step outside yourself and help you focus on things that are important to you.

Maybe it's your relationship, or the people around you.

Try writing about your day and keeping a record of how you feel, then read back over it when you're feeling stressed.

#11: Sleep More
And that's what I think is the most important step.

When you're feeling stressed, don't ignore your body.

Get in bed early, do some reading or meditation, and get a good night's sleep.

The effect of a good night's sleep is incredible, so make sure you catch some zzz's.

I would like to thank Lee from Science of Consciousness and Penny from The Universe is Trying to Tell Me Something for contributing to this post.

I also want to thank my therapist, Mariam Bolek, for providing the background for this post.

You Should Do Yoga Poses Every Day to Feel Great.

Mindful breathing is at the core of the practice—let your breath do the work. If you have to pause before breathing, notice that you're out of breath. Notice your breath is slower than usual. It's an opportunity to reset. Breath into your abdomen and blow air out. Bring your chest forward a little and breathe out. So now you're really relaxing into the full belly.

You'll also notice your heart rate is lower, and the physical sensations of exhaustion will decrease. Let your shoulders drop back and release the tension in your neck. Take a little time to rest, and notice how the pain from your shoulders and neck dissipates, leaving a much more spacious, spacious, spacious feeling in your body.

Anywhere you feel tightness, drop into a downward dog, resting your head back on a folded blanket or pillow. Exhale and breath in again and take your feet off the mat. Relax your neck and lift your chest. Breathe slowly, and let the tension of your upper back, neck, and jaw disappear.

Once you're ready, return to the pose, then take another moment to fully relax into the softness of your spine. Inhale, breathe out, and relax.

4. Solitude

On days when you're feeling heavy, try to be with yourself. Walk into a store, climb in bed, or do whatever else is at hand that you can do that will just be you and no one else. Take a minute and take a breath before you do anything else. Allow yourself that. Breathe.

Time for another mindful moment. Take a few deep breaths into your belly. This is where you'll release any stress you're carrying, and this is where you'll feel better. Now use that as a cue to just be quiet and peaceful for a few minutes. Notice your mind.

I highly recommend practicing through the day, even if only for a few minutes. It's good to get a whole series of gentle and restorative yoga poses done in one day. You'll feel rested and refreshed, and that's much better for you than leaving it till the next day.

5. Treat yourself

Are you a chocolate addict? Once you get some chocolate in your system, it can affect you, just like any other drug. If you can't stay away from it, at least make it a once a week treat. I used to buy my favorite chocolate bars in bulk and give them to friends, but I've since learned that it doesn't help.

When you get chocolate, eat it slowly. If you feel yourself salivating and you can't stop, swallow. It's best to stop now so you don't get into a routine. Consider a trail mix bar as a quick snack instead of a chocolate bar.

One final thought: Acknowledge that you're getting the calories you need—just in moderation.

Enjoy your meditation with some of the best breathing techniques and breathing for regular attention can significantly reduce your anxiety.

In today's chaotic world, anxiety is a very common problem. Meditation is a wonderful way to reduce anxiety in children.

Although parents can be too self-critical to allow the breathing action to penetrate the gray matter of their brain, children can reap the benefit of breathing and consciousness.

Meditation with children can help them to overcome stress and develop a greater sense of autonomy and confidence. Just sit with your child and get totally immersed in the breathing of the child to begin a meditative process for children as long as you can.

What should be taught during children's meditation?

We believe that you have to be present in the present moment to learn consciousness.

During meditation, we don't want to think about what else we want to or want to do.

Rather, we'd like to start to notice the physical breathing sensations.

While the breathing of your child is unchanged, try to get completely present at this time. You may begin to notice when the child begines to breathe more quickly or slowly.

Remember, if your child is stressed and anxied, the breathing will always feel uncomfortable.

A positive outcome of child meditation is that children start to feel the physical feelings of breathing – again. They begin to notice their breathing as something to like. Anxiety can slightly improve but react to constant disturbances in their environment.

Develop the meditation practice of your child

If your child is used to meditating with you, start this process from school days.

Let your child know, at least ten minutes, you will sit with them, do nothing but sit down with them and just breathe and look at them. Aske their questions as to how they feel, and leave their thoughts alone. Don't try to help them out.

Understand that some kids find this process difficult, especially if they're not used to sitting quietly.

It is a good idea to introduce longer meditation sessions into your daily routine. Some schools have also started integrating meditation into the curriculum.

If your child is reluctant to sit still, ask if during her free time she would like to do meditation in the gym. Or perhaps in the school cafeteria.

It is important for your child to be encouraged to develop this practice for her. Don't be harsh on the child.

Just be there and allow your child to follow her own path, you can't make her meditate, she must want to do it alone.

Don't wait for immediate results

The important thing is to start this process as soon as you can with your child. Make meditation a part of your daily routine.

If your child does not want to meditate at first, that's all right. Just let her choose other activities to stay entertained.

Recall that meditation isn't easy, it's highly demanding for the brain.

Children's meditation is not a quick fix, especially at an early stage. It takes patience and perseverance.

Your child will reap the rewards of meditation in the long term. More calm, more attention, a better sense of self-esteem and self-confidence.

Use patience

Try approaching your child kindly.

The aim is not to make your child meditate as soon as possible. We wish to help your child develop an attentiveness that can only be accomplished slowly.

For now, let her have her own way.

It is not easy to bond, especially during those tender years. Your child is always in a "guardian" state; instead of being a "teacher," she should see You as a caring mother.

Give your time to deal with your own emotions and learn to develop your own mental strength and resilience.

Seek professional assistance

If you worry about your child's possibility of a learning disability or a disability, make a doctor appointment, especially if your child is at school.

The doctor should undertake a thorough examination and give you advice and recommendations.

Your doctor will also be able to provide you with more information on how to involve your child in meditation.

Yoga is about firefighters' mental and physical health, emergency medical professionals.

Firefighter Joe Mastroleo, an 18 year-old paramedic, is an instructor on the Sunshine Skyway at the Fire Academy of Florida.

Mastroleo, 33, firefighter and paramédic of Pinellas County, told him he had decided to pursue a career as an instructor in 2015, when a colleague told him how important Yoga is to the first responders.

"Yoga isn't a dream. Yoga helps with stress management, and we have to make sure we're fully recovered if we're working 24 hours," Mastroleo said.

Other instruments used by firefighters include a five-day retreat program designed to train first responders in attention-care, stress management and healthy workplace coping skills..

Giafaglia said that retreat, which costs about $1,200 for firefighters who need it, helps participants to develop more self-confidence and self-regulation.

Mastroleo said that a cost-effective analysis based on research shows that he can reduce firefighter burnout by 50 percent by taking first respondents yoga or meditation courses.

One of the most important things firefighters can do for themselves and others is good mental health.

He said he acknowledges the techniques of stress management he learned at the retreat for his success as a paramedic and his ability to talk with patients in suicide.

Giafaglia said that he saw yoga and meditation capabilities to reduce stress and trauma and that such capacities are crucial to save lives.

"There are many links between trauma, burnout and suicide risks," he said.

Help on the Road

Starting this year, the United Way of Pinellas and Pasco counties received $5,000 from the Heart of Florida United Way in funding for a new First Respondent Suicide Prevention Program.

The deputy managing director of United Way of Pinellas and Pasco Counties, Mary Barstow, said that some of their funding will go to a job and training program for first responders interested in finding resources for mental health.

The Pinellas County Sheriff's Office works with United Way to identify those working with first responders and develop a program to help them cope with stress.

The aim, said Barstow, is to help first responders use their intuition to connect with needy people.

The United Way can reach people in need by different support groups, connect them to places where they can get help, and connect them to mental health and wellness organizations.

"We can connect you to a number of places to help you along the way," said she. "The goal is to get them trained on that side."

The two plans are only that, Barstow said – one for deputies and a second for paramedics.

Barstow said she hoped that two people would be part of the program and help others by the end of the year.

The Sheriff's office in Pinella County will work together with the United Way to get the program up and running. Mastroleo said the meditation training the burners receive from the Retreat also helps them to ask the right questions when they are dealing with suicidal people.

"The biggest thing we learned at the retreat is the way we can listen to these individuals and get the right information," said Mastroleo.

CEO of the Heart of Florida, Marty Lambert, said the organization is excited to offer the program in partnership with the Pinellas County Sheriff's Office and Pinellas County Fire Rescue.

He said there are many first respondents who work in the county of Pinellas and many of them deal with personal difficulties.

"We have seen many people who have struggled with many different things," said Lambert. "We wanted to address many issues to make sure they do well."

In summary, all about yoga, I want to tell you that it's the best thing you can do now for the sake of health. Even if you have lots of health problems, you should do yoga because it's like a powerful training that will help you to lose weight, to gain strength, to feel good, and to enjoy life as much as possible.

Enjoy your meditation with some of the best breathing techniques.

Yoga is about mental and physical health

Summarizing everything about yoga want to tell you that it's the best thing that you can do for you health now.

Enjoy your meditation with some of the best breathing techniques.

In today's chaotic world, anxiety is a very common problem. Meditation is a wonderful way to reduce anxiety in children.

Although parents can be too self-critical to allow the breathing action to penetrate the gray matter of their brain, children can reap the benefit of breathing and consciousness.

Meditation with children can help them to overcome stress and develop a greater sense of autonomy and confidence. Just sit with your child and get totally immersed in the breathing of the child to begin a meditative process for children as long as you can.

What should be taught during children's meditation?

We believe that you have to be present in the present moment to learn consciousness.

During meditation, we don't want to think about what else we want to or want to do.

Rather, we'd like to start to notice the physical breathing sensations.

While the breathing of your child is unchanged, try to get completely present at this time. You may begin to notice when the child begines to breathe more quickly or slowly.

Remember, if your child is stressed and anxied, the breathing will always feel uncomfortable.

A positive outcome of child meditation is that children start to feel the physical feelings of breathing – again. They begin to notice their breathing as something to like. Anxiety can slightly improve but react to constant disturbances in their environment.

Develop the meditation practice of your child

If your child is used to meditating with you, start this process from school days.

Let your child know, at least ten minutes, you will sit with them, do nothing but sit down with them and just breathe and look at them. Aske their questions as to how they feel, and leave their thoughts alone. Don't try to help them out.

Understand that some kids find this process difficult, especially if they're not used to sitting quietly.

It is a good idea to introduce longer meditation sessions into your daily routine. Some schools have also started integrating meditation into the curriculum.

If your child is reluctant to sit still, ask if during her free time she would like to do meditation in the gym. Or perhaps in the school cafeteria.

It is important for your child to be encouraged to develop this practice for her. Don't be harsh on the child.

Just be there and allow your child to follow her own path, you can't make her meditate, she must want to do it alone.

Don't wait for immediate results

The important thing is to start this process as soon as you can with your child. Make meditation a part of your daily routine.

If your child does not want to meditate at first, that's all right. Just let her choose other activities to stay entertained.

Recall that meditation isn't easy, it's highly demanding for the brain.

Children's meditation is not a quick fix, especially at an early stage. It takes patience and perseverance.

Your child will reap the rewards of meditation in the long term. More calm, more attention, a better sense of self-esteem and self-confidence.

Use patience

Try approaching your child kindly.

The aim is not to make your child meditate as soon as possible. We wish to help your child develop an attentiveness that can only be accomplished slowly.

For now, let her have her own way.

It is not easy to bond, especially during those tender years. Your child is always in a "guardian" state; instead of being a "teacher," she should see You as a caring mother.

Give your time to deal with your own emotions and learn to develop your own mental strength and resilience.

Seek professional assistance

If you worry about your child's possibility of a learning disability or a disability, make a doctor appointment, especially if your child is at school.

The doctor should undertake a thorough examination and give you advice and recommendations.

Your doctor will also be able to provide you with more information on how to involve your child in meditation.

Yoga is about mental and physical health

Firefighter Joe Mastroleo, an 18 year-old paramedic, is an instructor on the Sunshine Skyway at the Fire Academy of Florida.

Mastroleo, 33, firefighter and paramédic of Pinellas County, told him he had decided to pursue a career as an instructor in 2015, when a colleague told him how important Yoga is to the first responders.

"Yoga isn't a dream. Yoga helps with stress management, and we have to make sure we're fully recovered if we're working 24 hours," Mastroleo said.

Other instruments used by firefighters include a five-day retreat program designed to train first responders in attention-care, stress management and healthy workplace coping skills..

Giafaglia said that retreat, which costs about $1,200 for firefighters who need it, helps participants to develop more self-confidence and self-regulation.

Mastroleo said that a cost-effective analysis based on research shows that he can reduce firefighter burnout by 50 percent by taking first respondents yoga or meditation courses.

One of the most important things firefighters can do for themselves and others is good mental health.

He said he acknowledges the techniques of stress management he learned at the retreat for his success as a paramedic and his ability to talk with patients in suicide.

Giafaglia said that he saw yoga and meditation capabilities to reduce stress and trauma and that such capacities are crucial to save lives.

"There are many links between trauma, burnout and suicide risks," he said.

Help on the Road

Starting this year, the United Way of Pinellas and Pasco counties received $5,000 from the Heart of Florida United Way in funding for a new First Respondent Suicide Prevention Program.

The deputy managing director of United Way of Pinellas and Pasco Counties, Mary Barstow, said that some of their funding will go to a job and training program for first responders interested in finding resources for mental health.

The Pinellas County Sheriff's Office works with United Way to identify those working with first responders and develop a program to help them cope with stress.

The aim, said Barstow, is to help first responders use their intuition to connect with needy people.

The United Way can reach people in need by different support groups, connect them to places where they can get help, and connect them to mental health and wellness organizations.

"We can connect you to a number of places to help you along the way," said she. "The goal is to get them trained on that side."

The two plans are only that, Barstow said – one for deputies and a second for paramedics.

Barstow said she hoped that two people would be part of the program and help others by the end of the year.

The Sheriff's office in Pinella County will work together with the United Way to get the program up and running. Mastroleo said the meditation training the burners receive from the Retreat also helps them to ask the right questions when they are dealing with suicidal people.

"The biggest thing we learned at the retreat is the way we can listen to these individuals and get the right information," said Mastroleo.

CEO of the Heart of Florida, Marty Lambert, said the organization is excited to offer the program in partnership with the Pinellas County Sheriff's Office and Pinellas County Fire Rescue.

He said there are many first respondents who work in the county of Pinellas and many of them deal with personal difficulties.

"We have seen many people who have struggled with many different things," said Lambert. "We wanted to address many issues to make sure they do well."

Conclusion

Summarizing everything about yoga want to tell you that it's the best thing that you can do for your health now.
Even if you have lots of health problems, you should do yoga because it's like a powerful training that will help you to lose weight, to gain strength, to feel good, and to enjoy life as much as possible.

I hope, that you really enjoyed reading my book.

Thanks for buying the book anyway!